Sex Positive
TALKS TO HAVE
WITH KIDS

A guide to raising sexually healthy,
informed, empowered young people

Melissa Pintor Carnagey, LBSW

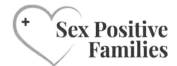

IN HONOR OF the powerful conversations that happen in homes every day, and for the parents and caregivers who deserve to feel better prepared for them.

ACKNOWLEDGMENTS

This guide was made possible by the collaborations and amazing expertise of: *Molly Platz*, digital designer; *Lisha Amin*, sexuality education consultant; *Ryan Horty*, editor; *Natalie Hatjes*, mindset coach; and *Ashley Gutierrez*, virtual assistant. Thank you for being a part of the dreamwork!

The unwavering support from Ryan, Aubrey, Tyson, and Owen is a lifeline to fulfilling SPF's mission. I'm so thankful for our love and family! I'm continuously inspired by you, Aubrey. You're my firstborn and reason for doing this work, so you, Tyson, and Owen have a better chance to thrive in your bodies, relationships, and sexual health journeys. It's truly an honor to walk this path of life together.

To my friends and colleagues who never fail to inspire with their brilliance, and who kept me from playing small in this process: *La'Toya Swan*; *Brittany Broaddus-Smith, LSW, MEd* (theintimacyfirm.com); *Dr. Lexx Brown-James* (lexxsexdoc. com); *Genia Jones-Hale* (createamagicalday.com); *Christie Federico* (christiefederico.com); *Goody Howard* (askgoody. com); *Dr. Donna Oriowo* (annodright.com); *and Cameron Glover* (cameronglover.com). Thank you for sharing your shine!

And finally, to the Sex Positive Families Instagram community, who is over 150,000 strong representing every identity and intersection from all over the globe (@sexpositive_families). You all are a constant reminder that fostering sex positivity in our families and communities is movement work, and we are not alone in this. Together we are creating safer, shame-free sexual health possibilities for the next generations, and connecting to healing for ourselves. Thank you for trusting me and this space.

TABLE OF CONTENTS

Dear Parents and Caregivers,

I'm so glad you're taking steps toward supporting the sexual health of a young person in your world. I'm Melissa Pintor Carnagey, a sexuality educator, licensed social worker, and parent of three young people (one of which is now an adult!). I know from both personal and professional experience the importance of opening up talks about topics like bodies, consent, sex, and relationships when raising empowered kids.

If you're feeling any bit nervous, overwhelmed, or unsure about what to share with your child and when, know it's perfectly normal to feel this way. This guide is designed to take away the guesswork and give you tools you can start implementing right away to support a child's sexual health and safety.

At Sex Positive Families, we believe, and research supports, that when young people have early and ongoing sexual health talks with caregivers, they make safer and more informed decisions in their life. This guide is perfect for parents and caregivers who want to provide the sex positive, shame-free foundation they wish they'd had growing up. I've included over 150 questions, reflection exercises, activities, and a wealth of resources to support you in the everyday talks with kids across ages. I want you to feel confident in your role as a sex positive mentor for your child. This guide will get you through.

As you dive in and start incorporating this content into your lives, you may have specific scenarios or questions that come up. Our website at sexpositivefamilies.com offers additional resources for every topic covered in this guide. You can also book a private coaching session to receive personalized support and customized resources from a sex positive parenting educator. I am here to support your journey!

I hope you enjoy this guide and find it a helpful tool along your path.

Keep up the loving work!

Melissa Pintor Carnagey, LBSW
Founder & Sex Educator

Introduction to Sex Positive Parenting

"In a society that profits off sexual shame, raising sex positive kids is radical, healing work."

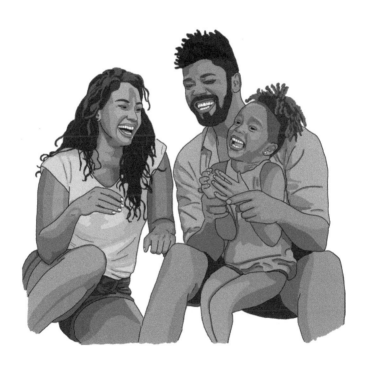

BEING A SEX POSITIVE FAMILY

Being a sex positive family involves more than talking about the birds and the bees. In fact, **moving away from taboos and moving toward open, honest, shame-free talks are what's necessary to become a sex positive family and create a solid foundation of sexual health for kids.**

Sexuality is an aspect of being human that is with us our entire lives, not simply a phase that starts at puberty. This means there are many opportunities within childhood to foster a young person's sexual health early and ongoing. From teaching accurate names for their genitals, to modeling consent in everyday life, sexuality education is about more than just sex and reproduction. It's available through teachable moments that begin before it's even about sex.

Some parents worry that if they talk about sex or sexuality with their kids, it will lead to early sexual behavior. Nothing is further from the truth. Research finds that when young people receive education and support specific to their sexual health, they are more likely to delay their first time having sex, use contraception when they do have sex, and be thoughtful about the number of sex partners they engage with. Talking with young people prepares them for informed decision making and lets them know you are a trusted adult they can turn to for support along the way.

Reflection: *When you think of your own upbringing, how comfortable did you feel talking about bodies, relationships, and sex with adults in your world? What influenced this comfort level?*

But, won't the schools teach them about this stuff?

I wish we could count on this. The sad reality, especially in the United States, is that schools are falling short when it comes to sexuality education. At the time of this publication, only 28 states and the District of Columbia mandate sex and HIV education in public schools. Furthermore, only 17 states require the content to be medically accurate. Sounds wild, right?!

Our young people receive all levels of math- more than they will ever use in their adult life- but are shortchanged when it comes to learning about their bodies, consent, healthy relationships, and sexual decision making. These are vital life skills. It's for these reasons that families must play an active role to ensure young people are prepared, not scared, along their journeys.

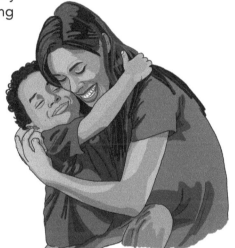

The more confident and equipped parents are for sexual health talks, the safer, more informed young people will be. **Informed kids grow into empowered and prepared adults. I believe parents are key influencers in leading them there.**

WHAT IS SEXUAL HEALTH?

According to the World Health Organization, **sexual health is a state of physical, mental, and social well-being in relation to sexuality.** It's more than just sex and encompasses many aspects of the human experience.

Take a look at this word cloud, which includes topics that fall under the umbrella of sexual health. As you use this guide, consider which topics you wish to explore further on your own and which topics you plan to talk about with a child in your world.

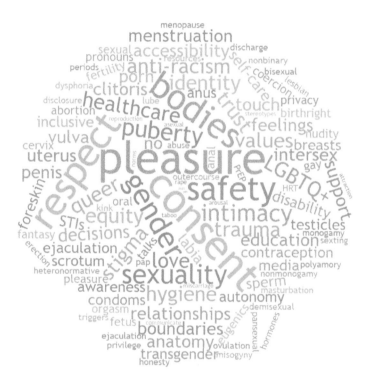

What other sexual health topics, not represented in the word cloud, are important for you to learn more about or discuss in your family?

_____

_____

_____

_____

STARTING THE TALKS

Why does talking with kids about sexual health feel so challenging?

I'm frequently asked about the best way parents and caring adults can show up for the talks without feelings tripped up or avoidant. These topics can feel tricky for many adults today for several reasons:

- **Growing up without open talks about sexual health**
- **A lack of quality comprehensive sex education, which just was not offered (and still isn't) in many schools**

- **Being raised within purity culture or under religious belief systems that shamed or erased sexuality**

- **Having an identity that is systemically oppressed, hypersexualized, objectified, or de-sexualized by society-particularly Black, Brown, Indigenous, LGBTQ+, fat, and disabled folx**

- **The influx of social media and streaming porn-- influences we did not encounter as kids**

- **Experiencing sexual trauma, consent violations or policing of the body, at any point along your sexual health journey**

All of these factors are real and can take time to work through. It's important to know that none of these are your fault. When I entered parenting over 20 years ago, I did so as a Black and Latinx 17-year-old who grew up within a Catholic-influenced culture. We did not talk about sex or sexual health at home, and I certainly wasn't getting informed in Texas public schools. I'd experienced my share of trauma and consent violations, knew the impact it had on my own sexual health and wanted to do better for my children. I've had to employ lots of self-compassion along the way to undo generational traumas and the habits that were not serving me in building the kind of relationship with my kids that keeps them safer, more informed, and empowered. **Showing up for sexual health talks along the journey has been a key element to successful sex positive parenting.**

HOW TO RESPOND

Though there isn't a perfect script when talking to your child about sexual health, there are some steps you can take to open the dialogue and better navigate their curiosities, with less awkwardness.

1. DON'T PANIC!

Hearing questions from young kids like, *"What is sex?"* or *"Where do babies come from?"* or *"Why does my penis do this?"* can cause discomfort or an urge to avoid the subject. We want to get to a place where talking about bodies, identity, consent, relationships, and sex is as normalized as talking about the weather. How we react to a child's curiosities can influence whether they continue to come to us. Any questions they bring your way are a sign that they see you as a safe space and trusted resource. For this, give yourself a high-five.

2. RESPOND IN AN AFFIRMING WAY

A good go-to response is: *"That's a great question! I'm so glad you asked."* Using affirming statements reassures a child that their curiosities are always welcome, no matter the topic they bring to you. This is critical, especially when we are working to build the kind of trusting connection that makes them more likely to speak up if anything unsafe or concerning happens.

Alternatively, if we respond to a child's question with silence, changing the subject, or if we flat out shut them down, it sends them the message that these topics are not welcomed. This is the beginning of shame. When it comes to sexual health, even in the face of the most seemingly 'awkward' or 'sexualized' curiosities, you want to make sure they know that no topic is taboo.

3. GET CURIOUS (NOT INVESTIGATIVE)

So you've established with your child that you appreciate their question, now send a curiosity right back their way. Something like, *"What have you heard about sex?"* or *"What do you think it means when your penis does that?"*

Not only does this give you a few more moments to gather your thoughts, their response can offer more context that helps frame the information you offer next. Who knows, maybe they meant something totally different than you assumed? For example, "Where did I come from?" might not be a question about reproduction or sex, but simply wondering in what city they were born. Asking might also lead to you learning that their question was influenced by a concerning situation or experience that needs your follow-up.

You'll want to avoid any accusatory or investigative questions that can cause a child to feel like they're being punished, attacked, or shamed. Steering away from questions that begin with *"Why..."* is one way to minimize this.

4. FIGHT THE URGE TO RUN

You're not on fire! If it feels like you are, that's completely normal. Take a breath. You've got this! Remember that this is a teachable moment. Avoiding it can send the message that asking these kinds of questions is not okay, which can shut them down in the long run. You both have an opportunity for growth and connection through the experience. Don't hesitate to acknowledge any discomfort, so it isn't interpreted incorrectly by your child.

5. ANSWER THE QUESTION

You've stuck this moment out. Now you want to answer the question. Keep some considerations in mind, such as their age, unique personality, and the setting you're in at the time. The information you give a six-year-old will be different than the information you would give a teenager. Some kids love detail and long talks, while others lose interest quickly. As such, your response can be anything from simple to scientific to anecdotal. You can choose your own adventure in the way you wish to connect and support your child's curiosity.

What if I don't know the answers?

Kids have amazing, limitless curiosities as they're searching for meaning in their world. You won't always have all the answers. Any information you're unsure of, you can look up together or let them know you will get back to them. Then make sure you actually do.

The Sex Positive Families website offers links to hundreds of resources-- books, videos, podcasts, webinars, toys-- that help you to be a responsive adult. Remember, our children are not wanting us to be encyclopedias. They want us to be present, available, and supportive when they need us.

What if my kid doesn't want to talk about this stuff?

Each young person is unique, so these conversations are more effective when they don't feel forced. Using pressure will only shut them further down.

These topics are not inherently awkward, but sometimes in our homes or communities we make the topics feel that way by how we react when issues related to bodies, consent, or sex come up. Our children pick up on this early and they adapt. This can create a learned discomfort and avoidance. To talk openly about taboo topics, they have to feel safe to be able to ask questions or receive information, without worry of being judged or punished for it.

If you're getting resistance or being shut out when trying to talk about sexual health, some good old vulnerability and honesty is one way to influence a shift in direction. It can sound like:

> *"I realize that I haven't always been as open as I've wanted to with you about important topics like bodies and sex. That has a lot to do with how I grew up. I didn't have someone teaching me about these things or making me feel safe to talk about them. I want to provide you with a more open experience, so you know you can come to me if you need to, and that it's totally normal for you to have questions about these things. It's okay if this moment doesn't feel like the best time. I'm going to get some books for our house, so we have resources here. I might check back in with you again soon. If you want to talk anytime, just let me know. I'm feeling more prepared. Thank you for being patient with me on this."*

Acknowledging where you've been and where you'd like to go together in terms of the talks is a great way to set the intention for the actions to follow. In a statement like this, you're also making it clear that you're not forcing the conversations.

Find casual moments to spark a no-pressure chat, like when you're riding in a car together or on a walk or as related topics come up in something you're watching together. You'll likely notice a shift in how they react and relate to you. See it as one opportunity of many more ahead.

SETTING THE TONE

The earlier you start with an open, shame-free approach, the more relaxed the conversations about sexual health will be with young people. So, if you're reading this while raising littles, you have a great opportunity to set a taboo-free tone now. These topics aren't inherently awkward or uncomfortable; they become that way if that's how they're introduced to a child.

If you're reading this as a parent of older kids, you might have just winced. But don't worry, it's never too late to foster a more open dialogue. It takes some patience and consistent follow-through to establish the trust needed for your young person to see you as someone they can turn to, when discussing these topics.

Consider these ten tips when setting the tone for shame-free, sex positive talks:

1. YOU WERE YOUNG AND CURIOUS BEFORE, DON'T FORGET THAT. Think to yourself, what support did I need when I was their age? When we disconnect from that vulnerability, we become less empathetic and approachable to our child.

2. FOCUS ON PREPARING THEM, NOT SCARING THEM. Be careful not to focus your conversations on risks or fear-based messaging. See every talk as an opportunity to prepare them with the skills and awareness to lead satisfying sexual health journeys.

3. LISTEN TO UNDERSTAND, NOT TO RESPOND. This is especially important as they get older. This guide is full of great open-ended questions you can use to invite their perspectives.

When they answer them, just listen. Don't rush to give advice, jump to conclusions, or have all the answers.

4. BE HONEST. They can tell when we're feeding them bullshit or when we're trying to keep information from them. If they're old enough to have asked, they're old enough to receive an honest response.

5. RESPECT THEIR AUTONOMY. Instead of trying to control their outcomes and decisions, accept and honor their right to self-determination. Get comfortable with asking, "What do you think about that?" and "How can I support you?"

6. WALK THE TALK. It's the most effective way to earn a young person's trust. If you want them to respect others' boundaries, have a positive body image, understand healthy relationships, or express their feelings, you've got to consistently model it yourself. If you're working on things, be honest with them about that. Give them the space to work on things too without expecting perfection.

7. KEEP THE LEARNING FUN. Thankfully, there are so many options now for introducing or deepening sexual health knowledge. From podcasts to pop-up books, interactive apps to animated videos, sex education isn't the same boring stuff we may have seen growing up. Engage them in ways they like to learn, and be open to try new resources.

8. MINIMIZE JUDGMENT. If your child senses that they will be teased, punished, or silenced for being curious, they will be less likely to engage with you. It doesn't mean they're not wanting to know this stuff. They just know not to go to you about it. If you want more openness, ask yourself- how am I making it safe for my child to talk to me about these topics?

9. DON'T ACT LIKE YOU KNOW IT ALL (BECAUSE YOU DON'T). Get comfortable with saying things like, "I don't know. That's a great question. Let's look that up together." If you hold onto pride, you risk losing credibility and their trust. It's also valuable to model not having all of the answers, and learning how to seek them out.

10. **KEEP AN OPEN DOOR.** The goal is to have lots of little conversations over time, not just one, and every talk is an opportunity. Let your child know that you're always there for their questions or concerns. Nothing is off-limits, weird, or too much. Make it clear that your primary role is to be a trusted support to them, no matter what comes their way.

> **Reflection:** *How comfortable do you want your child to feel talking with you about their sexual health questions and concerns? What steps are you taking to make that possible?*

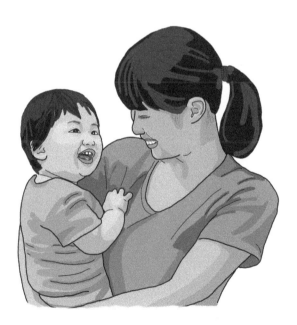

Conversation Starters by Age

"Raising sexually healthy children is the opportunity to be the caring adult you needed."

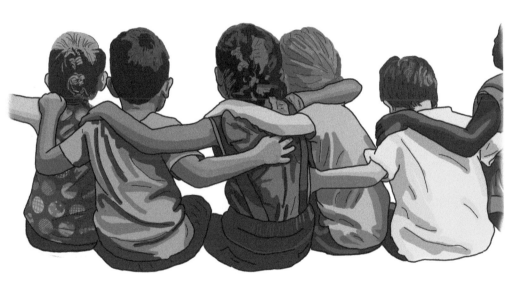

Body Awareness

LET'S TALK ABOUT BODIES

MENSTRUATION TALKS, PERIOD.

GETTING REAL ABOUT FEELINGS

MASTURBATION (A NOT SO TOUCHY SUBJECT)

LET'S TALK ABOUT BODIES

When children know their bodies, they develop the awareness that keeps them safer and better equipped to advocate for their needs and boundaries. It's important that parents feel comfortable talking about bodies, so let's do a little challenge to see where you're at on this.

How many of these words can you communicate without laughing, lowering your voice, or wincing?

- [ ] Arm
- [ ] Nipple
- [ ] Ear
- [ ] Elbow
- [ ] Clitoris
- [ ] Vagina
- [ ] Penis
- [ ] Testicle
- [ ] Scrotum
- [ ] Vulva
- [ ] Breast
- [ ] Anus

How did you do? If you noticed a difference in your reactions to the words that society tends to correlate with sex, versus the non-sexualized words, that can be a sign that you've internalized certain messages that can affect your comfort level when thinking or talking about these body parts. If that's the case for you, hold compassion versus shame. Many of us grew up in homes and within education systems that did not normalize bodies or provide accurate information. The great thing is that you are now able to create better possibilities for a child in your world.

You can take this challenge steps further by adding other terms for body parts or sharing the list with different family members or friends to see how they do and what conversations are sparked as a result. Practice until there's no hesitation, taboo, or shame.

Conversation Starters

Birth to Age 3

"This is an ear. This is an elbow. This is a penis. This is a vulva."

"I bet that felt good to get that pee/poop/fart out. Your body did it's job! Let's get you changed."

Using accurate words for all body parts, especially genitals, gives children the language that keeps them safer and informed. Talking to infants through diaper changes and bathing gets you both in the habit of using correct terms in shame-free ways.

It's also important to normalize bodily functions early. Children learn, through the reactions of others around them, ways to interpret the natural processes of their body. If others laugh or say "eww" when their body relieves itself, it becomes a habit they follow and sends an underlying message of shame or embarrassment. These reactions can follow people into adulthood, making it difficult for people to experience natural bodily functions without feeling the urge to hide or hold judgment. Consider how your family talks about and reacts to bodies, so you're consistent about the messages you wish to send.

TIP: *The next time you sing, Head, Shoulders, Knees, and Toes add some genital anatomy terms to make it sex positive.*

Ages 4 to 8

"Our bodies have many jobs that keep us healthy. Let's talk about what penises and vulvas do and how people take care of them."

"It's so important that we get to know and respect our body, especially the parts that we usually keep private behind clothes. Let's do an activity that helps us learn more about genitals."

This age is perfect for teaching about the functions of genitals, how to clean and care for them, the importance of privacy when enjoying the pleasures of self-touch (masturbation) as well as recognizing unsafe touch. Activities like using play dough to create the parts of their genitals, using paper and colors to make art that celebrates their body, or reading a book about bodies together, all can stimulate the talks in fun ways.

TIP: *Check out the Sex Positive Families' website Resources section to find age-congruent options that work for your family.*

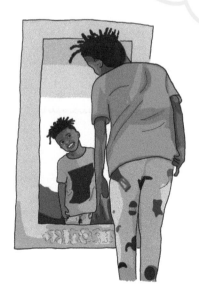

Ages 9 to 12

"You may start to feel and see changes in parts of your body or hear your friends talk about it. What do you know about puberty?"

"It's common to wonder, Is my body normal? Remember that bodies are uniquely designed and all bodies are good bodies. If you ever have questions about your body, let me know so I can help answer them."

"It's a good idea to get familiar with how your unique genitals look, feel, and even smell. This can help you tell when anything seems different or worrisome."

Tweens, no matter which genitals they have, will start to notice changes happening to their body. Keeping an open dialogue is the best way to prepare them for greater confidence.

When they know they can come to you or another trusted adult, it keeps them connected and safer. If you'd like support and a safe space to learn about puberty with other families, check out our website for virtual puberty workshops and courses.

TIP: *Encourage your tween to get to know their body. A handheld mirror can be a great tool to allow them to check out the parts that are harder to see.*

Ages 13 and up

"Let me show you the steps for scheduling a doctor's visit and when it may be needed for your sexual health."

They're growing up! As they begin to transition to adulthood, help them learn when and how to see a medical provider for annual exams, STI testing, contraception, reproductive, and mental health.

Reflection for Parents & Caregivers

Take a moment to reflect on the following questions (either on paper, internally, or with another caregiver), to consider how your own personal values, experiences, and knowledge impact how you approach conversations about body awareness, with your young person.

How comfortable are you using medically accurate words for genitals?

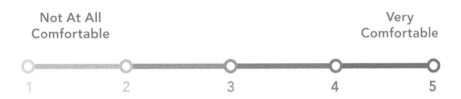

Not At All Comfortable   Very Comfortable

1   2   3   4   5

What personal experiences have influenced your comfort level?

_____

_____

_____

_____

_____

What would you like your child to understand about their body? About all bodies?

_____

_____

_____

_____

_____

MENSTRUATION TALKS, PERIOD.

Young people of all genders need to know how menstruation works. This helps them develop a shame-free understanding of bodies, people with uteruses, and reproductive health.

Whether or not you are someone who menstruates, and regardless of the level of knowledge you have at this moment about periods, you can start the talks that keep children informed and better able to apply their knowledge in positive ways toward supporting their body and the bodies of others.

If you're not sure how menstruation works, here's an inclusive rundown of the process:

- Starting in adolescence, people with uteruses can bleed for a few days monthly. It is natural. It's not dirty or wrong. It happens when an ovum (one of thousands of eggs that people with uteruses are born with) is not fertilized by sperm.

- Sperm is the other half of what creates a human baby. Sperm is made in the bodies of people with testes. An ovum and sperm cell can meet during some types of sex or with the help of a doctor.

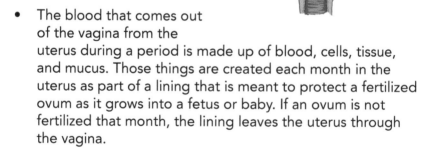

- The blood that comes out of the vagina from the uterus during a period is made up of blood, cells, tissue, and mucus. Those things are created each month in the uterus as part of a lining that is meant to protect a fertilized ovum as it grows into a fetus or baby. If an ovum is not fertilized that month, the lining leaves the uterus through the vagina.

- It can take around 3-7 days for all of the lining to exit and generally does this process monthly, as long as an ovum is not fertilized.

- Some people use menstrual products like pads, a cup, tampons, and period underwear which collect the blood when it exits, instead of the blood landing on clothes.

- During menstruation a person can feel other things like cramping, bloating, or changes in mood because the body is working hard and doing amazing things.

It's important that people who are menstruating are supported and respected. The depth of the information you share with a child can vary by age, curiosity, and their cognition level. There are many amazing, fun resources nowadays to support these talks.

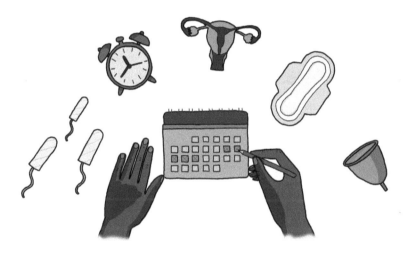

Check out the Menstruation section of the Sex Positive Families' website to find additional resources that will engage your family.

Conversation Starters

Birth to Age 3

At this age it's not only about what you say, but what you do. If a person in the home menstruates, opportunities can arise monthly to normalize and create positive visibility around this bodily process. That can look like:

- Not hiding the fact that period products (ex. pads, menstrual cup, tampons, period underwear) are in the home

- Taking a child down the menstrual care aisle in a grocery store to show them what some options look like and what they're used for

- Being open about the ways a person who menstruates can be supported during their cycle, and allowing your child to help out (e.g. allowing the person who menstruates to get more rest or bringing them a fresh menstrual product)

- Answering- versus avoiding- questions a child might ask if they notice signs that an adult in their life menstruates

The earlier menstruation is acknowledged, without shame or secrecy, the more natural it remains to talk about as the years move forward.

Ages 4 to 8

"Menstruation, also called a period, is when blood leaves the body through the vagina for a few days each month. It happens to people who have a uterus and is a pretty amazing process. Let's read a book or check out a video to learn all about how it works."

Around the preschool years, it's common to field many curiosities about bodies. Instead of hesitating or worrying you might say the "wrong" thing or give too much information, use an age-congruent book or engaging video to support the talks. It can provide a fun way for kids to learn about menstruation and also takes the pressure off of you to know exactly what to say and when.

TIP: *Check out the Menstruation section of the Sex Positive Families' website to find our favorite resources for this age group. Pick one to use today to begin or further the talks.*

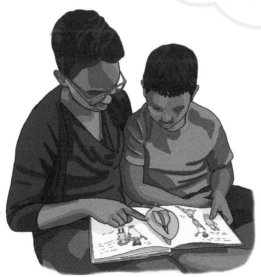

Book Pictured: "Vaginas and Periods 101: A Pop-Up Book" by Christian Hoeger & Kristen Lilla

Ages 9 to 12

"You/Your friends might be having periods now or in the near future. It's a natural part of puberty for bodies with a uterus. Have you noticed these changes happening? What would you like to know more about?"

As puberty starts to show up for a tween and their peers, it becomes so important that they are prepared to know what to expect, how to react, and what resources are available for support. This could include talking more in depth about what truly happens within each cycle; exploring the different menstrual health products available; or creating or purchasing a first period kit.

If your tween has a uterus, you want to make sure you're having this discussion before the bleeding begins, so they're prepared, not scared. For talks with tweens who don't have a uterus, you don't want to avoid the topic. These conversations can create a foundation for tweens to serve as supports to peers and others in their life who menstruate.

For trans or nonbinary young people with a uterus who do not identify with stereotypical femininity or girlhood, having periods can contribute to feelings of gender dysphoria. Opening up the talks lets your young person know you are an affirming support. Trans teens may be interested in pursuing puberty blockers to assist their body in better aligning with their gender identity. If this is the case, talk with a trans affirming primary care doctor or therapist. The Human Rights Campaign has information to help parents locate resources near you.

Ages 13 and up

For teens with a uterus, menstruation can either be in full swing, may not have started, or is infrequent. A parent's best role is remaining an open, shame-free support. This can look like:

- *Ensuring the home is regularly stocked with period products* of the teen's choice or if they're a non-menstruator with menstruating friends, keeping products in the bathroom for when guests visit can be a thoughtful gesture

- *Not speaking negatively about menstruation or puberty symptoms*; not allowing anyone in the home to either

- *Checking in with menstruating teens each month* about how their period has been going or whether they've experienced any concerning changes with their body

- *Assisting a teen, in ways they find helpful,* for medical checkups or reproductive health appointments

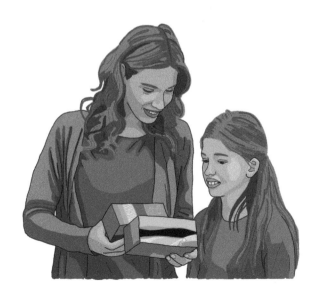

Reflection for Parents & Caregivers

Take a moment to reflect on the following questions (either on paper, internally, or with another caregiver), to consider how your own personal values, experiences, and knowledge impact how you approach conversations about menstruation, with your young person.

How was the topic of periods and menstrual cycles treated in your home or community growing up?

_____

_____

_____

_____

_____

How comfortable do you feel talking to a child about menstruation?

Not At All
Comfortable   Very
                                          Comfortable

O———————O———————O———————O———————O
1   2   3   4   5

What would you like them to understand about periods?

_____

_____

_____

_____

_____

GETTING REAL ABOUT FEELINGS

When children learn to identify, express, and trust their feelings, as well as recognize the emotional responses of others, they develop the skills that support body awareness, safety, and overall wellness. As a child grows, these skills become vital tools for fostering healthy relationships and safer, mutually satisfying experiences into adulthood. The education begins early and can be learned through everyday activities and discussions, before it's even about sex.

One easy activity you can use to explore feelings is to play a feelings scavenger hunt. Here's how it works:

While watching television, movies, or YouTube videos that depict people interacting, mute the sound and/or remove captions. Together, observe the facial expressions and body language of the people in each scene then take turns pointing out what emotion you each think the person is experiencing.

Are they happy, excited, scared, sad, angry, frustrated, lonely, embarrassed or another feeling? How can you tell?

Then take it a step further and ask questions like:

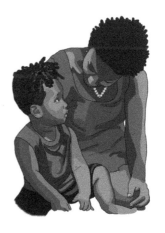

- When was the last time you felt that emotion?

- What was going on?

- What did that emotion feel like in your body?

- If it felt like a difficult emotion, what did you need to help you through that feeling?

- When you notice someone experiencing that emotion, what can you do to support them?

This activity is a fun way to help children develop the language and awareness of self and others, that keeps them safer and more confident communicators.

Conversation Starters

Birth to Age 3

"I'm feeling frustrated right now because..."

"I am excited about going on a walk today!"

"I am worried we might be a little late, but I know we will get there soon."

Parents can help lay the foundations for a child's understanding of feelings, by staying connected and open about their own emotions and modeling how to communicate them with others, so children learn first by example.

Ages 4 to 8

"What does it feel like in your body when you are scared/happy/mad/sad/excited?"

"What do you think they are feeling right now? How can you tell?"

As children's communication abilities increase, find ways to help them express what they are feeling. What they see others feeling. These skills support safety, foster empathy, and are building blocks of giving and receiving consent.

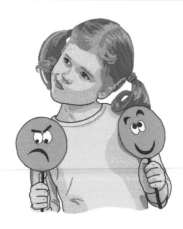

Ages 9 to 12

"Your body is going through big changes to get you through puberty. What have you noticed?"

"Some changes are physical and some are emotional. At times it might feel amazing and other days, not so much. That's totally normal."

"When I was going through puberty, I remember feeling _____."

"If you need extra support along the way, I want you to know I'm here for you. I will do my best to be available and understanding."

The shifts in hormone levels that tweens can experience during the puberty years can contribute to some fluctuating and challenging emotions. The best thing you can do is be present and affirming. These talks can also create a perfect opportunity to reflect and share about your own puberty journey. This fosters empathy and connection.

Ages 13 and up

"I'm here to listen."

"How best can I support you?"

Simple but powerful phrases that honor the autonomy of teens and make clear that you're still an available touchstone on their path, as needed. Making a judgment-free space for their feelings means we engage in more listening and less fixing.

Reflection for Parents & Caregivers

Take a moment to reflect on the following questions (either on paper, internally, or with another caregiver), to consider how your own personal values, experiences, and knowledge impact how you approach conversations about feelings, with your young person.

Growing up, how affirming of your feelings were the adults in your world?

_____

_____

_____

_____

_____

How did these early experiences impact you?

_____

_____

_____

_____

_____

_____

What skills related to feelings do you hope to foster for a child in your world?

_____

_____

_____

_____

MASTURBATION
(A NOT SO TOUCHY SUBJECT)

Pleasure is an integral part of being human. When young people establish trust in their bodies as a safe place to explore and experience pleasure, they're better prepared for safer, more satisfying experiences along their journey.

To get them there, it's important children understand that their bodies:

- Are uniquely designed
- Have an array of amazing functions
- Require routine care for wellness
- Are theirs to decide how they wish to be touched and by whom
- Can experience wonderfully pleasurable, soothing sensations

These truths begin as early as in the womb and exist throughout their lifetime. Supporting their body awareness means reassuring your child that touching their body is natural, not wrong. That if they ever have questions about their body, feel pain or discomfort, experience an unsafe moment or person, or need help with their body, that you (or another trusted adult) are available to talk to.

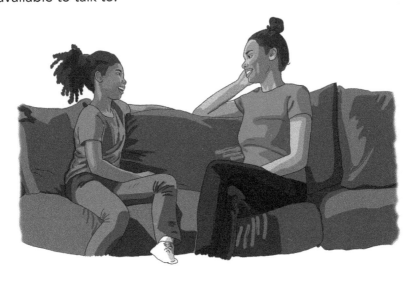

Conversation Starters

Birth to Age 3

It is perfectly natural for infants and toddlers to explore their bodies, especially their genitals. It's not adult eroticism or a direct sign of abuse. It often means the child is aware of their genitals' capacity for pleasure, which are packed with thousands of nerve endings. It can also mean the child feels safe and comfortable in their environment. Supporting the foundations of body trust and pleasure means caregivers do not shame or punish young children when they explore their bodies.

Ages 4 to 8

"I notice you're touching your penis/vulva/genitals/anus. If it's itchy or hurting, tell me, so I can help."

"It can feel good to touch our own genitals. We do this in private. We're at/in the [name the non-private place] right now, so it's not a private place. If you want to enjoy more touching, you can go to [name of private space]."

During the elementary years, children are better able to understand privacy and social norms related to touching their genitals, and can apply this awareness to respect communicated boundaries. Gentle redirection and reminders can be used when needed, to minimize shame, while still affirming that self-pleasure is a natural experience.

Ages 9 to 12

"Masturbation can be a positive way to get to know your own body- what feels good to it and what does not- before you invite anyone else to."

Whether a tween chooses to masturbate or not, it's important that they develop a taboo-free connection with their own body. This better ensures that they're not reliant on another person for their pleasure, and that future partnered sex, if they choose to engage in it, will involve greater self-awareness and confidence. This ultimately keeps them safer.

TIP: *Check out the Pleasure section of the Sex Positive Families' website to find resources that support talks about masturbation.*

Ages 13 and up

Parents have asked me what they should do if they walk in while their teen is masturbating. My answer is: apologize for not knocking first, and walk back out of the room.

Give a teen their space and privacy to explore their own body and sexuality. This maintains the respect that will keep them trusting you as someone they feel safe to turn to when support is needed.

Reflection for Parents & Caregivers

Take a moment to reflect on the following questions (either on paper, internally, or with another caregiver), to consider how your own personal values, experiences, and knowledge impact how you approach conversations about masturbation, with your young person.

How was the topic of masturbation handled when you were growing up?

_____

_____

_____

_____

_____

What are your values related to masturbation?

_____

_____

_____

_____

_____

What would you like your child to understand about masturbation and self-pleasure?

_____

_____

_____

_____

_____

Consent and Safety

CONSENT-CONSCIOUS CHATS

Consent is a life skill that should be practiced long before it has anything to do with sex. When we seek consent before moving forward with an action, we are acknowledging another person's right to their own choice in an experience. We're acknowledging that permission is required to move forward with an action.

As we receive the response, the important next step is that we respect and adhere to the wishes and boundaries of another, without being dismissive or coercive. This process is a foundational aspect of consent.

Families can create a consent-conscious home by using this approach in many different ways within daily interactions. For example:

- *"May I take a picture of/with you?"*
- *"Would you like a hug?"*
- *"Can I have a bite of your snack?"*
- *"Is it okay if I tell ___ what you shared with me?"*
- *"Would you like help with that?"*
- *"They said stop, so that's enough. No one says 'no' or 'stop' more than once before the boundary is respected."*
- *"May I post this picture online for others to see?"*
- *"Can I borrow your...?"*
- *"No? Okay, I respect that."*

Some may argue, *"why do I have to ask permission from a child?"* or *"they're MY child, and until they're on their own in the world, they do what I say."* Thoughts such as this are what gets children accustomed to being controlled by another, operating out of a sense of obligation, and less able to assertively communicate their needs without fear. It essentially grooms them to be victims or oppressors within abusive relationships.

Some exceptions are when children are in stages of earlier development or if they're living with disabilities that require adults to make decisions on their behalf. In those cases, the leading phrase before an action is performed may sound more like, *"I'm going to...,"* as a way of walking through intentions with open communication. Paying attention to non-verbal cues is absolutely important, being ready to make adjustments or stop as needed in response.

When we don't seek consent, we assume another person's feelings, wants, and needs. We send the message that our will and desire is more important than theirs.

Raising children who become adults that understand consent and healthy boundaries means creating a home culture where the necessary skills and communication are consistently practiced, long before it has anything to do with sex.

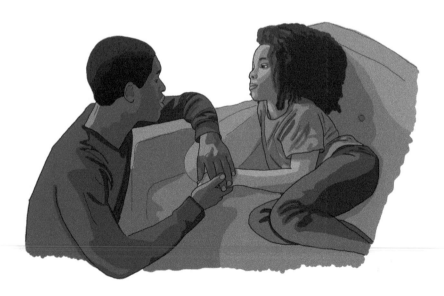

Conversation Starters

Birth to Age 3

"Please ask before you touch my child. Consent is important to our family"

Before a child is communicating on their own with the world, they need caregivers who can model setting boundaries that honor their bodily autonomy and safety. Reminding strangers and others that consent and respect is important in the early years is one step.

Ages 4 to 8

"You are the boss of your body. If you ever do not want to share affection or don't want someone to touch you, let's practice what you can do and say..."

When children understand their rights to bodily autonomy and practice the options available for setting boundaries that feel comfortable to them, we prepare them for confident, safer interactions with others. Together, you can practice the many options for greeting people, if hugs or kisses are not desired, such as waving, saying hello, giving a high-five, shaking a hand, fist-bumping, or smiling.

Make sure you're clear, and teach them that adult feelings do not override their safety. If another adult tries to bargain or coerce them into receiving unwanted touch, this is not the behavior of a safe adult. Even if it's a family member, talk about what steps they can take to prioritize their safety and how to disclose when something uncomfortable or unsafe occurs.

Ages 9 to 12

"Respecting the consent of other people isn't just about listening for a 'no.'"

It's critical children know that consent is also about affirmative yeses, paying attention to the body language of others, and must be voluntary and conscious. This education starts well before they're making decisions about sex.

TIP: *Check out the Consent resources on the Sex Positive Families' website to find books, videos, games, and webinars that help your family explore the nuances of consent.*

Ages 13 and up

"What are some of your boundaries related to sex and relationships?"

"Have you ever been in a situation where someone did not respect your boundaries? What did that feel like? How did you handle the situation?"

When teens know their values and limits, they can make decisions with greater confidence and less contradiction. Making a shame-free space to talk openly about what they do and don't want in these areas, and ways to communicate with partners, helps them to be prepared.

Reflection for Parents & Caregivers

Take a moment to reflect on the following questions (either on paper, internally, or with another caregiver), to consider how your own personal values, experiences, and knowledge impact how you approach conversations about consent, with your young person.

How consent-conscious was your own upbringing?

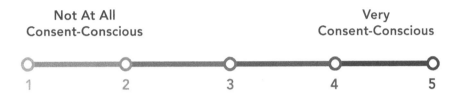

Not At All Consent-Conscious				Very Consent-Conscious
1	2	3	4	5

In what ways has this influenced your experiences with setting and receiving boundaries and consent?

_____

_____

_____

_____

_____

What would you like your child to understand about consent?

_____

_____

_____

_____

_____

BEING OPEN ABOUT SAFE AND UNSAFE TOUCH

Talking with children about safe and unsafe touch prepares them to trust their instincts and to recognize the signs of untrustworthy people and situations.

One frequent question I receive from parents relates to how to respond to children playing doctor or wanting to touch each other's genitals. Children being curious about their own genitals and the genitals of others are both very common aspects of sexual development. Their curiosity and desires to explore do not make them sexual predators or deviant. When we truly understand this, we are better positioned to respond from a place of confidence versus fear or shame.

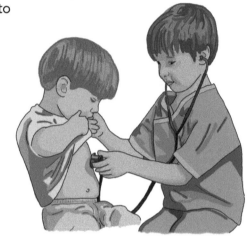

A general rule of thumb is if kids have an age gap of three or more years, they are no longer considered within each other's peer group and the risk is high that an inequitable power dynamic is involved. This makes them more vulnerable to unsafe touch or coercion. This also applies if one or more children have a cognitive or developmental disability or neurodiversity. Consent must be informed and that cannot happen with children as they are not able to understand what they are truly consenting to or effectively advocate for their body boundaries.

When addressing instances of genital exploration between kids, use clear phrases and gentle redirection. For example, *"We don't touch their penis/vulva/genitals. It is a sensitive area. It's okay to be curious, but we want to be safe with each other. Let's read a book about bodies so you can learn more."* Help them to learn under what circumstances genital touch from others during childhood is appropriate (e.g. for help with hygiene care by trusted adults, when needed, or during medical care) and how they can speak up when they are uncomfortable or feel unsafe.

Children may seek out body exploration or genital touch with another child even after you've addressed it once with them, so consistent messaging and follow-up is key. Create spaces that minimize the risk of recurrence, such as ensuring there is trusted adult supervision during play; that you're offering consistent reminders; and, you're providing them with ongoing education about consent and body safety.

If you suspect that sexual abuse is a factor in what is influencing a child's behavior, follow your gut. It is true that children who have experienced sexual trauma, especially if it has gone unaddressed, can act out sexual behaviors as a result of their trauma. So if you have any doubts, a couple great organizations to reach out to for support are *rainn.org* and *stopitnow.org*. They have hotlines available and resources that can help caregivers ensure they are taking the appropriate next steps to support all involved.

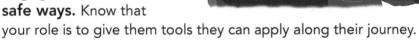

Children need the guidance of caring adults to help them understand how to engage with others in safe ways. Know that your role is to give them tools they can apply along their journey.

Books, videos, and conversations about situations that arise can all be great ways to integrate education about consent, body safety, and safe/unsafe touch. Check out the Resources section of our website to find options for your family.

Conversation Starters

Birth to Age 3

"Show me your body bubble!"

Play can be a great time to engage toddlers in exploring concepts of privacy and boundaries. To support the learning, try the body bubble game. Invite the child to use the tip of their finger to draw an invisible bubble around their body. They can reach as high, low, or wide as they want to. They can even imagine the colors or designs of their bubble. You do the same by drawing yours. Then walk around the room together, and anytime someone gets close to each other's bubbles, make a sound.

This offers a chance to practice creating and respecting body boundaries. Talk about times when using a body bubble can be helpful (like in new places or around new people) or times when the child feels comfortable inviting someone they trust into their bubble, like for a hug, and who those people in their life might be. Remind them that, at any time, they can change the shape of their bubble and set a different boundary.

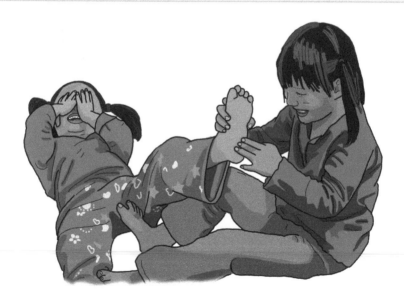

Ages 4 to 8

"What does it feel like for you when you feel safe? What does it feel like when you don't feel safe?"

"No one is allowed to touch or ask to see your genitals. If you are sick or hurt, a doctor might need to examine your body, but they should always talk to your trusted adult first and let you know what they are doing. You have the right to say no or stop at any time. It should be respected."

"Let's think of three adults you trust. These are people that if anything unsafe were to happen, you'd feel comfortable telling them and you know they would help you stay safe."

"If you ever need to share that something unsafe has happened, I will believe you. You will not be in trouble."

It's important to explore concepts of safety with a child early- what it feels like to be safe; which situations or people are trustworthy; what they can do in an unsafe situation; and who they can turn to for support. These talks, like all others, should be ongoing and integrated into everyday moments. You can use age-congruent books or videos to keep the learning engaging and fun.

Ages 9 to 12

"Have you ever been in a situation or with a person that you didn't feel safe or comfortable with? What about that situation or person made you feel this way? What can you do if you're ever in a situation like that again?"

Our growing tweens will enter more situations where we aren't right by their side. Helping them develop a critical lens, stay connected to their instincts, and devise next steps will keep them safer and supported along their path.

Ages 13 and up

"What are you looking forward to most today/this week?"

"How are things with (partner or friend) going right now?"

"I want you to know that if you ever need an ear or someone to talk through difficult situations with, I'm here for you."

The teen years are where developing new relationships, sexual experimentation, and risk-taking can take place. Find the opportunities to stay connected with what is going on in their world, including what and who are most important to them. It's a chance to be an available touchstone, versus an investigator or gatekeeper, which gives them space to explore their own values, goals, and experiences while still knowing they have your support when needed.

Reflection for Parents & Caregivers

Take a moment to reflect on the following questions (either on paper, internally, or with another caregiver), to consider how your own personal values, experiences, and knowledge impact how you approach conversations about safe and unsafe touch, with your young person.

What ways are you keeping a brave space for a child to come to you if they have concerns or need to disclose an unsafe situation?

_____

_____

_____

_____

_____

If you are a survivor of sexual abuse or trauma, what supports are you engaging to nurture your healing journey?

_____

_____

_____

_____

_____

What skills would you like your child to develop when it comes to understanding safe and unsafe touch?

_____

_____

_____

_____

Identity Development

TALKING ABOUT GENDER

EXPLORING TALKS ABOUT SEXUAL ORIENTATION

TALKING ABOUT GENDER

Many of us were socialized to view gender as binary identities limited to two options- girl/boy or woman/man. The truth though, is that gender exists on a spectrum, so the possibilities are far more vast and diverse. To understand the nuances, it helps to break it down into **gender identity, gender expression, and sex assigned at birth.**

Gender identity is how a person thinks of or identifies themselves relative to gender. Examples are girl/woman, boy/man, femme, transgender, nonbinary, genderfluid, and genderqueer.

Gender expression is the physical representation of a person's gender through things like their clothing choices, hair, or personal style. From a binary lens, it can relate to how feminine or masculine a person presents, but it can be a mix or neither of these. Examples of terms related to gender expression are feminine, masculine, androgynous, neutral, conforming, and nonconforming.

Sex assigned at birth, also referred to as biological sex, is a label given when a person is born and often is based on an assessment of their external genitals. Examples of these terms are female, male, and intersex. Intersex people can be born with genitals, chromosome patterns, internal organs, or hormone levels that fall outside of what's typically categorized as female or male. Because of these varying factors, that aren't always visible at birth, a person may not learn they are intersex until puberty or later in life or may never find this out about themselves.

Check out the glossary on p.97 for more vocabulary.

Understanding gender and the different ways people can identify, express themselves, and how bodies can develop is an important part of staying open and affirming to the beautiful diversity that exists.

How a person expresses their gender can change and is not up for debate by others. It's best that parents and caregivers allow young people to explore how they identify and like to express themselves without placing limits or expectations.

To learn more about gender, check out the *The Gender Unicorn*, an educational graphic created by the Trans Student Educational Resources (TSER).

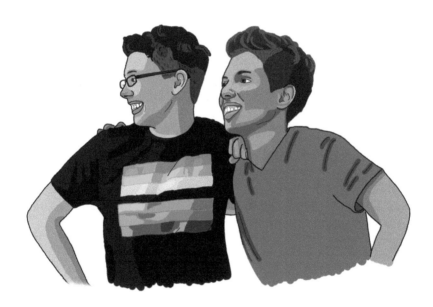

Conversation Starters

Birth to Age 3

From the time a child is born, they are receiving messages from the people and world around them about gender identity, gender roles, and gender expectations. For this reason, the first few years of life are a great time for caregivers to explore what has influenced their attitudes, beliefs, assumptions, stereotypes, and experiences related to gender. This includes considering the ways your family intends to uphold or challenge gender constructs.

Ages 4 to 8

"Colors, toys, and clothes can be for everyone, not just boys or girls. Which colors, toys, or clothes are your favorites? Which would you like to try out?"

When children can enjoy things they are interested in, and are taught to respect others' choices, they can develop more expansive ways of expressing themselves and appreciating others' individuality, without limits based on gender.

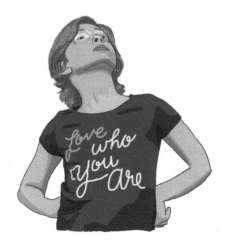

Ages 9 to 12

"People can receive messages about how they 'should' look or behave based on their gender. What do you think about this? What are some examples of messages you've received before?"

Young people take in many messages about gender from peers, school, media, the internet, and adults, which can influence their developing identity and decisions. Opening up a space to consider what these messages mean can help them explore their own identities and to develop a critical lens about the outside influences that shape their experiences with gender.

Ages 13 and up

"I'm grateful to have you in my life."

"I respect you."

"I love the ways you express who you are."

"You inspire me."

The identity exploration continues in the teen years and on into adulthood for many. What young people need most, no matter how they identify, is a clear sense of the support they have from the people that matter most to them. Alongside using affirming words, make sure your actions align with the message. Abandon a desire to critique or control. Instead, give them the space to explore and thrive in their unique identities.

Reflection for Parents & Caregivers

Take a moment to reflect on the following questions (either on paper, internally, or with another caregiver), to consider how your own personal values, experiences, and knowledge impact how you approach conversations about gender, with your young person.

What messages or expectations did you receive about gender growing up?

_____

_____

_____

_____

_____

How did these messages shape your perceptions of your own identity and how you expressed yourself?

_____

_____

_____

_____

What would you like your child to understand about gender?

_____

_____

_____

_____

EXPLORING TALKS ABOUT SEXUAL ORIENTATION

A person's sexual orientation is:
- Theirs to explore
- Theirs to disclose (if they ever wish to)
- Not up for debate
- Not determined by others (including a parent)

Sexual orientation, like gender, exists on a spectrum and can be fluid. Many times it's based on physical or emotional attraction toward particular gender identities, but it also can be defined by not experiencing physical or emotional attraction at all.

Sexual orientation does not always correlate with whether a person is having sex with another person or whether a particular event has occurred between people of certain gender identities (e.g. dating, engagement, marriage, cohabitating, or raising children together). And there isn't a particular way that a child or adult acts that defines their sexual identity; only that person can (or can choose not to) define it for themselves.

> Some of the frequently discussed sexual orientations are heterosexual or straight, gay, lesbian, and bisexual, but there are many more. Other examples include:
>
> - **Aromantic**   - **Asexual**   - **Demisexual**   - **Pansexual**

If any of these identities are unfamiliar to you, check out the Glossary of Terms at the end of this book, or head to our website's Resources section to explore more.

A caregiver's most effective role is in being open and available to be supportive of their child no matter which gender identities they may or may not feel sexual or romantic feelings for. This means not making assumptions about which genders a young person will have feelings for and not placing expectations on a child's future as it relates to their relationship status or life goals. Instead, follow their lead and be prepared to support their developing identities as they move through adolescence into adulthood.

Conversation Starters

Birth to Age 3

Reflection: *What values do I want to share with my child as they grow, that will influence their understanding of attraction and love?*

This is a reflective question to explore on your own or with other caregivers in your world so you create a supportive home culture early.

Ages 4 to 8

"There are many different ways that people can be a family together. Our family includes [insert your dynamics - e.g. two moms, a dad, two children, and a cat], but that's not the same for all homes. Have you noticed that? What are some examples of different types of families you've seen?"

It's common for children to notice differences in the people and world around them. These observations can be used as early teachable moments about the beautiful diversity of relationships, attraction, and families. Fostering respect and acceptance for the many ways love can be experienced helps them see the possibilities that exist for their own futures as well.

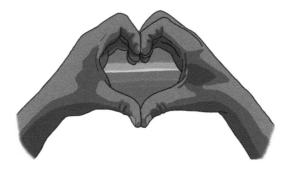

Ages 9 to 12

"People can use words like lesbian, straight, gay, bisexual, asexual, and pansexual to express who they feel attracted to."

Talking openly about different ways people can express and experience attraction to others can help normalize feelings they and peers around them may be having. Never force another person to choose or disclose their sexual orientation. Sexual orientation, like gender, exists on a spectrum and can shift throughout a person's life.

TIP: *If any terms are unfamiliar to you, use the glossary at the end of this guide and dive into the Sexual Orientation section of the Sex Positive Families' website to learn more.*

Ages 13 and up

"Your happiness, as you define it, is important to me."

"I'd love to get to know more about your date/partner. What do you like most about them?"

"I support you."

Remember, a young person's sexual orientation and who they grow to love (if anyone) is not for parents or others to dictate. For LGBTQ+ youth especially, familial rejection can lead to riskier behaviors and impacts to their mental health. Unconditional support is what all youth deserve and need from family. Show genuine interest in their lives and the people that mean the most to them. Give them the space to explore and thrive as their most authentic selves without fear or shame.

Reflection for Parents & Caregivers

Take a moment to reflect on the following questions (either on paper, internally, or with another caregiver), to consider how your own personal values, experiences, and knowledge impact how you approach conversations about sexual orientation, with your young person.

Growing up, what representations of different sexual orientations did you experience?

_____

_____

_____

_____

_____

How have these experiences influenced you?

_____

_____

_____

_____

_____

What would you like your child to understand about sexual orientation?

_____

_____

_____

_____

_____

Intimacy

GETTING REAL ABOUT RELATIONSHIPS
THE SEX TALKS

GETTING REAL ABOUT RELATIONSHIPS

Talking to children about what it means to have healthy relationships prepares them for safer, mutually pleasing, and respectful connections with others.

A great activity to explore on your own, is to make a list of the qualities or features of a healthy relationship. Ask yourself, what does a healthy relationship feel like when you're in one? What do the people involved do, not do, say, or not say that makes it healthy? See how many ideas you can come up with. You can take it a step further and place a star next to the top five or ten features that you feel are essential. Think about why you feel that way. Reflect on whether you've experienced any of these qualities before, and within which relationships in your life those have occurred.

What you also may find yourself thinking about are qualities of an unhealthy relationship. Feel free to make a list of those as well. Doing this activity, though simple in its design, can sometimes stir up challenging memories or emotions. Be gentle with yourself.

The final step is to look at one or both of these lists, and think about what a person needs in order to be able to recognize or maintain these features of a healthy relationship. It's in this that we can identify what skills we can help foster and model for a young person in our life, so they have the opportunity to know what to look for, and that they're clear that they deserve that much, along their path.

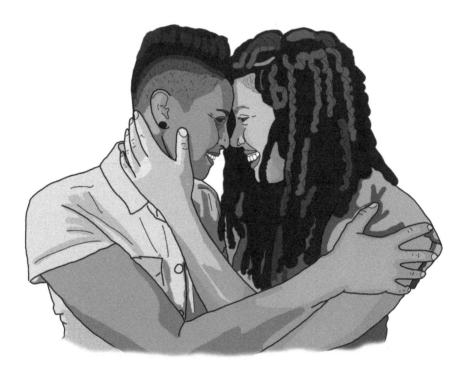

Conversation Starters

Birth to Age 3

Reflection: *In what ways am I modeling behaviors of healthy relationships? In what areas could our household or family improve?*

Like it or not, actions speak louder than words. A child's primary education on relationships comes from what they observe and experience from the interactions within their own home. Use these reflective questions to explore, on your own or with other caregivers in your world, your existing strengths or challenges in modeling healthy relationships.

Ages 4 to 8

"Who's a friend that you like spending time with?"

"What makes them a good friend?"

"How can we show a friend that we care about them?"

Early friendships are the training ground for understanding how to interact with others in loving, respectful, and safe ways. Sibling relationships also offer up many opportunities to explore these elements. Before a child enters into their teens or adulthood, help them build awareness of the qualities and behaviors that keep relationships feeling good to everyone involved.

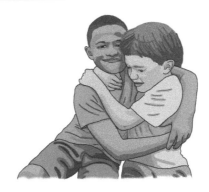

Ages 9 to 12

"What does a healthy relationship look and feel like? What about an unhealthy one?"

Relationships come in many forms from friends, family, professional connections, and intimate partners. Talking through the ingredients of a healthy relationship can help young people also explore signs of an unhealthy relationship. Knowing the difference can keep them safer and more prepared for the road ahead.

Ages 13 and up

"When I was a teen, I thought relationships were _____. I wish I'd been told _____."

Sharing aspects of your own experiences with topics like relationships can be a powerful way to connect with teens. Even if your path has included relationship fails or difficult moments, the wisdom you've gained from them can be a valuable resource for teens trying to make sense of their own situations and decisions. Remember that you get to decide how much or what to share. You may find that they're more willing to open up to you when you model vulnerability with them.

Reflection for Parents & Caregivers

Take a moment to reflect on the following questions (either on paper, internally, or with another caregiver), to consider how your own personal values, experiences, and knowledge impact how you approach conversations about relationships, with your young person.

What type of relationship dynamics did you grow up seeing in your home?

_____

_____

_____

_____

_____

How did these experiences influence your understanding of relationships?

_____

_____

_____

_____

What would you like your child to take away from conversations with you about relationships?

_____

_____

_____

_____

_____

THE SEX TALKS

I connect with thousands of parents and caring adults each year in this work, and a common reflection expressed is the poor-to-no sex education they received growing up, and the impacts it has had on their journeys. Though we can't go back in time to change our own experiences, we can absolutely influence more informed opportunities for the next generation.

Shifting the narratives for our kids doesn't mean we abandon talking about contraceptive options, condoms, or STIs, it just means that we don't limit or center the conversations to just those topics. That we stay open to talking about all types of sex (e.g. oral sex on all genitals, anal sex, fingering, hand jobs, dry humping, mutual masturbation, sex using toys) not just the kind of sex that can lead to pregnancy. And we speak honestly about the fact that sex is most often for pleasure.

When young people are not informed that sex should be both pleasurable AND consensual, they're not adequately prepared with the necessary communication, awareness, and interpersonal skills that best ensure their safety and satisfaction within a sexual encounter.

When parents deny, dismiss, or erase pleasure, it contributes to a higher probability that their young person finds themselves:

- Faking orgasms
- "Consenting" to sex when it isn't truly desired
- Feeling shame toward their own body and sexuality
- Not being aware of and confident within their own body
- Being less aware of the non-verbal cues of partners
- Not knowing how to communicate about their wants, needs and limits
- Being victims or perpetrators of sexual assault or abusive relationships

When young people are ill-informed and under-prepared, they cannot make informed choices or notice the signs of an unhealthy dynamic. They are far less able to be responsive to changes within their own body.

Conversations about sex are not about birds and bees; they're about humans, bodies, pleasure, and consent. The foundation for these talks begin early and can help young people feel clear about who the resources and supports are for honest, accurate, and shame-free information about sexual health.

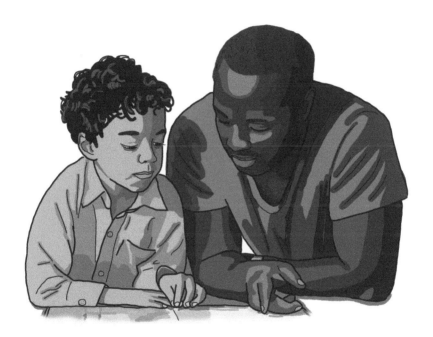

Conversation Starters

Birth to Age 3

Reflection: *How did you learn about sex? What is your definition of sex? What or who has influenced your understanding of sex?*

Well before you're having talks with children about sex, they are taking in messages about sexuality from the adults in their world. Creating a home culture where sex talks are not awkward or shame-based begins with you. Use these reflective questions to take inventory of the values and influences that have informed your understanding and beliefs about sex.

Ages 4 to 8

"Let's talk about where babies come from."

In the early years it's common for kids to be curious about reproduction, especially if they have a new sibling arriving or begin to notice pregnant people. This is a great time to share facts, in direct responses that they can understand, which lay the foundation for later talks about sex. Creating openness early is what will keep them feeling safe to return to you as a trusted, shame-free support.

TIP: *Check out the resources within the Sex Positive Families' Reproduction section on the website, for fun, age-congruent options to support the talks.*

"It's perfectly normal to be curious about sex. If you ever have any questions, I am happy to give you an honest answer. If it's something I don't know, we can look it up together with a trusted resource."

"What things have you heard or learned before about sex? What questions do you have about sex?"

"You might hear people talk about virginity or first time sexual experiences. Let's talk about what this really means and what a person can expect when having sex for the first time."

Normalizing curiosities about bodies, relationships, and sex is an important part of fostering a taboo-free home culture. Young people are more likely to turn to their parent or primary caregiver if they can trust that they won't be shamed or judged for asking questions. There are many angles to approach the topic; the tween years are a great time to take the talks a bit deeper, share your values, before they rely on information from peers, online searches, or porn.

When you talk about sex, make sure you're not limiting the conversation to one type of sex. Ensure you're talking about the importance of communication, consent, and pleasure for all involved, and that you're not focusing solely on avoiding STIs or unintended pregnancy.

Ages 13 and up

"Let's talk about ways to stay safer, if and when you choose to have sex."

"The first time you touch a condom or dental dam, shouldn't be the first time you're having sex. Let's run to the store and pick up some barrier methods, so I can show you the steps for using a condom correctly."

"Have you put any thought into what barrier methods or contraception you or a partner may need? If you'd like help exploring the options, I'm happy to talk this out and do some research with you"

These are the sex talks that early conversations have been building up to. Help them think ahead about contraceptive options, barrier methods (like condoms or dental dam), sexually transmitted infections, consent, pleasure, and how to talk about all of these areas with a partner. Be careful not to limit the information based on your assumptions but to create a nonjudgmental space. The goal is to prepare, not scare, them.

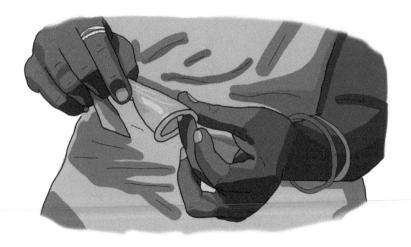

Reflection for Parents & Caregivers

Take a moment to reflect on the following questions (either on paper, internally, or with another caregiver), to consider how your own personal values, experiences, and knowledge impact how you approach conversations about sex, with your young person.

What is something you wish you'd been taught about sex?

_____

_____

_____

_____

_____

What does being sexually healthy mean to you?

_____

_____

_____

_____

_____

What would you like your child to understand about sex?

_____

_____

_____

_____

_____

Media Literacy

FOSTERING MEDIA LITERACY

Keeping children safer online takes more than setting up parental controls. It involves fostering ongoing talks that help a child develop a critical lens for media's influence, so they have the skills to make safer and informed choices. These skills create conscious consumers of any form of media, whether it's print, YouTube, video games, social media, apps, movies, music, or the news.

Media literacy skills help children:

- Think critically about the media they take in
- Become not just conscious consumers, but also conscious creators
- Appreciate varied perspectives and points of view
- Understand the role of media and the internet
- Make informed choices about how to engage with media and while online

Like all other topics, the talks and education begin early and can be fostered through everyday teachable moments. This best ensures that young people are prepared to make sense of what they may see, hear, feel, and what messages come their way.

Conversation Starters

Birth to Age 3

Reflection: *When and how do I want to introduce devices to my child?*

It's not uncommon for children in infancy to first interact with electronic devices, so it's important to assess early your family's agreements around usage. This is a reflective question to explore on your own or with other caregivers in your world so you create a supportive home culture early.

Ages 4 to 8

"Who do you think this message was made for? What tells you that?"

"Who created this? What tells you that?"

"Why did they make it? How can you tell?"

"What details were left out? Why do you think they were left out?"

"Who was represented and who was left out? Why do you think it was created this way?"

"How did the content make you feel?"

"Would you recommend this to someone you care about? Why or why not?"

Media literacy is about an ability to critically evaluate content- it's intended audience, purpose, creator, meaning, credibility, and how it made you feel. Through thoughtful talks that can begin in the early years, children can develop skills to become safer and more conscious media users. These questions can be integrated into everyday conversations as you consume media together, until they become a part of a child's inner dialogue.

Ages 9 to 12

"What do you enjoy about using a [cell phone, tablet, computer, gaming system]?"

"What do you like to use your device(s) for?"

"How much time each day would you like to be able to use your device(s)?"

"Let's work together to name each of our screen time wants, needs, and limits. Then we can come up with some agreements that work best for our family."

Screen time limits are one protective measure that can support a young person's safety and media literacy until they are able to manage it more effectively on their own. Every family is unique, so when considering how to create limits on device usage, involving everyone in the process creates buy-in and gives a space for people to communicate their concerns, ask questions, or advocate for what's important to them.

Once you've established agreements, consistency is key, but also keep in mind that it's perfectly okay to identify a test period, try it out, then come back together to share how it went. You can always make changes together and establish new agreements as needed.

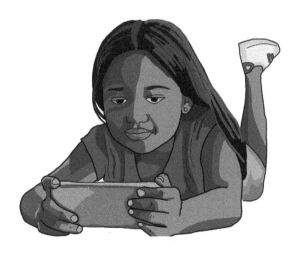

Ages 13 and up

"What are your opinions about social media? Do you feel it does more good, more harm, or does it depend?"

"What's the biggest challenge you've faced while being on social media or online?"

"Have you ever been bullied or treated badly online? Have you ever seen this happen to someone else? How did this feel? How did you handle the situation?"

"Let's talk about the importance of creating a digital footprint you can feel confident in."

Whether your teen is on social media or not, it's a high traffic virtual playground for young people. A lot can go on there in a short period of time, so it's important that you keep open communication and a welcoming space for them to share how they're engaging on the web. The more awareness and support they have, the better equipped they are to make informed and safer choices while online.

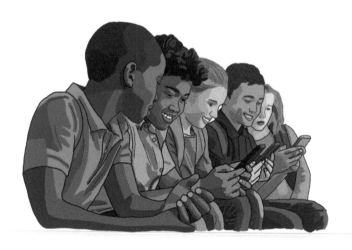

Reflection for Parents & Caregivers

Take a moment to reflect on the following questions (either on paper, internally, or with another caregiver), to consider how your own personal values, experiences, and knowledge impact how you approach conversations about media literacy, with your young person.

What messages did you internalize as a result of the media you consumed growing up?

_____

_____

_____

_____

_____

What limits, boundaries, and agreements does your family have in place when it comes to screen time?

_____

_____

_____

_____

_____

What would you like your child to understand about media literacy?

_____

_____

_____

_____

_____

HONEST TALKS ABOUT PORNOGRAPHY

Young people today have cell phones, devices, apps, gaming, web browsers, and social media at their fingertips and at earlier ages than ever before. Whether it's their own device, one of a parent (often handed over to "occupy" them), or the device of a peer, their access points are many and are often unfiltered.

Preparing children for sexual health and safety is more than trying to block or limit access. We must:

- Engage them early in conversations that build their awareness, critical thinking, autonomy, and informed decision making around the body, relationships, consent, and sex

- Listen and observe, with a focus on learning and connection, not control

- Be as accessible to them as online porn is

It's about mentoring more than it is about monitoring or micromanaging.

If we don't create open, shame-free spaces for their curiosities to land, they will more likely turn to risky experimentation, peers, or online porn. Creating an open dialogue about online porn and sexually explicit media, can safeguard young people from unsafe situations.

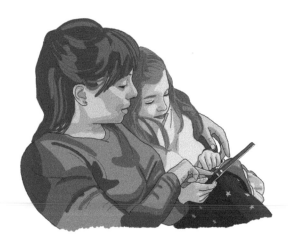

Conversation Starters

Birth to Age 3

Fill in the blanks:

I believe online porn is _____.

I believe online porn is not _____.

The best ways to safeguard young people from early exposure to online porn are _____.

Talks about online porn won't happen with an infant, but taking a proactive approach involves assessing your own attitudes, values, assumptions, and feelings about online porn. Use these fill in the blank statements to reflect independently or with a partner or fellow caregiver to explore your thoughts on this topic.

Ages 4 to 8

"If you ever come across pictures or videos of people naked or touching each other's genitals or private parts, this is called pornography or porn. These images are for adults not kids. If you see things like this, you're not in trouble, but I'd like for you to turn off the device or step away from it and let me or a trusted adult know so we can help explain what you've seen."

With the prevalence of online porn access by young people, it's important to be clear early about what they should know and do about a situation where they've been exposed to sexually explicit media. Remaining silent on the issue, leaves them more vulnerable to unsafe or confusing situations. Opening up the dialogue in a shame-free way makes it clear that you are a trusted adult they can turn to for support.

TIP: *Check out the Pornography section of the Sex Positive Families' website as well as the Tackling Talks about Porn webinar to learn how to have these conversations with greater ease.*

Ages 9 to 12

"It's normal to be curious about bodies and sex. Porn is not a safe place to learn about these things. If you ever have questions, you can come to me, but if you don't feel comfortable for any reason, let me show you some reliable, safe online places and resources that will answer questions you might have."

The tween years typically bring about specific curiosities about bodies and sex. This increases the chance that they, or a close peer, will go seeking out answers online. Google doesn't judge young people for wondering, and even with the best parental controls and filters, young people often find a way to get the information they seek. When parents and caregivers normalize their curiosities and provide pathways for youth to exercise their autonomy in safe ways, it often lessens their impulse for secrecy or thrill-seeking.

Ages 13 and up

"What's shown in the porn that you can find free online is not a realistic or fair representation of bodies, relationships, and sex. It's made for entertainment and to make money, and is often not ethically produced. It's important that you know this, so you don't enter into sexual situations thinking you or your partner have to act like or look like what you might see in porn."

Talking openly and proactively with teens about porn's influence, as well as its often inequitable and harmful representations of people and sex, can help them make safer decisions within their own sexual relationships. This can be an opportunity to talk about the true diversity of bodies, sexual consent, healthy communication, trust, respect, pleasure, safer sex practices, contraception, mainstream versus ethical porn, and sexual identity. As they enter adulthood, if they choose to consume porn, they'll be better equipped to do so consciously and view it as entertainment, not as a representation of sex off screen.

Reflection for Parents & Caregivers

Take a moment to reflect on the following questions (either on paper, internally, or with another caregiver), to consider how your own personal values, experiences, and knowledge impact how you approach conversations about pornography, with your young person.

What role did sexually explicit media or pornography play within your adolescent years?

_____

_____

_____

_____

_____

What is your comfort level in talking with your child about this topic?

Not At All
Comfortable

Very
Comfortable

O———————O———————O———————O———————O

1   2   3   4   5

What would you like your child to understand about sexually explicit media and online porn?

_____

_____

_____

_____

_____

WHICH TALKS WILL YOU HAVE TODAY?

I invite you to start somewhere. Pick one conversation starter and let it lead your family into deeper, shame-free connections. Make this content what you need it to be to support your sex positive parenting goals.

As you do, remember that **tackling these talks isn't about following a script or saying one "right" thing. It's about fostering a shame-free connection and being the caring adult you needed growing up.**

I believe in the power of your influence. You deserve to feel confident and better prepared for the conversations that will raise sexually healthy, informed, and empowered kids.

If you get stuck or need some backup, head to our website at sexpositivefamilies.com. There you can search resources by topic and age, catch a webinar, or book a private session to receive one-on-one support that'll get you through your next steps.

Thank you for being a valuable part of the SPF community and for trusting me along your path. Together, we are creating safer, more liberated possibilities for generations ahead. Keep up the loving work! This world needs us.

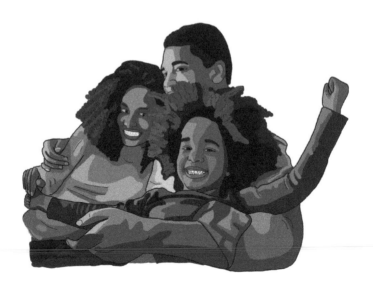

Resources and Support

"Knowledge is power, and we want young people to be really powerful!"

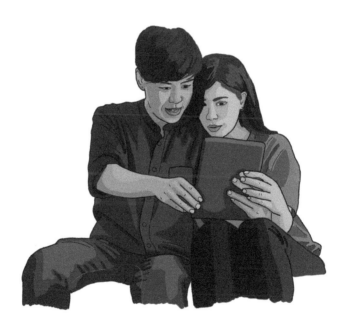

FREQUENTLY ASKED QUESTIONS

Q   *How do I talk to an autistic or disabled child about these topics?*

All young people need support and guidance along their sexual health journeys, so they know what to expect, how to take care of their bodies during changes, ways to stay safer, and who to turn to with questions. This is especially important for young people who have autism and/or a cognitive disability, who without an awareness of these big changes, could feel more alarmed, which makes it harder for them to adjust. They also can become more vulnerable to abuse or unsafe situations, without the skills to recognize what has occurred and what to do next.

When approaching the talks with children who have autism or a cognitive disability, consider the following:

- How do they like to learn new things? Is it through watching, listening, talking, playing a game, writing, movement, or creating art? Find creative ways to introduce these topics that align with their learning style. You can read a book together, play a board game while talking, color or draw, sing a body safety song, use playdough to craft anatomy, or watch an educational video.

- Consider when the best opportunities are within their day for connecting on important topics. Non-busy, laid back moments are typically best so there's not a sensory overload.

- Keep your expectations realistic and flexible. Don't place unnecessary pressure on them or yourself to cram in a lot of info in one talk, or to feel like they have to "get it" all the first time. The key to all sex positive talks with kids, is to explore topics through many different small conversations and interactions that can build on each other over time.

- Avoid lecturing. Keep the information and terms at the level they can understand.

- Don't assume they won't understand a topic. Introduce it as it feels relevant and watch for verbal or nonverbal cues that let you know whether they are comprehending or if it's time to move onto something else.

- Ask them, *"What do you think about that?"*, *"How does hearing that make you feel?"* or *"What questions do you have about this?"*

- Use resources with diverse representation, so they're more likely to see aspects of themselves as they learn. Check out our website at sexpositivefamilies.com/resources to search available options for each stage.

- Be sure to loop in other trusted adults, caregivers, or providers in their world. Keep an open dialogue with them about the importance of your child's sexual health education and how each person is working to support it. Always trust your gut if ever someone or a situation is not feeling aligned or safe with your child's sexual health and safety.

Q *Should girls and boys be separated when learning sex education?*

Inclusive, comprehensive sexuality education offers young people of all genders the opportunity to learn about sexual health. Separating kids by assumed gender can:

- Send a message that what happens to the bodies of others unlike them, should not be their concern or is a secret

- Perpetuate a false narrative that there are only two gender identities and only two ways genitals and internal anatomy can develop

- Force young people to have to choose a (gender) side or have it chosen for them

- Fail to address the fact that gender and genitals are not the same

- Erase the experiences of transgender, gender non-binary, and intersex youth

- Rob young people of the opportunity to learn how to talk openly about sexual health with others who may have different bodies and identities than them

- Inhibit empathy, understanding, and shared knowledge

- Leave young people with unanswered questions about the sexual health of all bodies

In all of my years of teaching gender inclusive classes, one thing is very clear—Young people can absolutely handle and participate in education about all bodies and all genders. They consistently bring amazing curiosities about experiences and identities unlike theirs, when given the safe space to ask. That experience should not be held back from them. Most often the separation by assumed gender is crafted to pacify misguided assumptions and discomforts of adult decision makers or educators, not the youth.

Q   *I'm a survivor of sexual abuse and sometimes it feels hard to answer my child's questions or respond to things that happen on these topics because it can feel triggering. What can I do about this?*

Parenting in a sex positive way can feel triggering, scary, daunting, or unclear if you did not grow up with positive experiences related to these topics. They can trigger unpleasant memories and unexpected feelings of fear or loss. Because sexual health is often treated as taboo, being triggered by these topics can also feel isolating, with few safe spaces to talk about it and find clarity.

Hold lots of compassion and patience for yourself. Take notice of any moments where you have a triggered reaction or you feel big shifts in your body. If you need to pause and take a few breaths, that's always a good way to ground yourself and give nourishing oxygen to the brain. Reach out for support, whether that's a partner who can step in to help or listen; a therapeutic space that allows you to process what's coming up and practice new coping strategies; or connect with parent groups for survivors, so you stay reminded that you're not alone.

While parenting in a sex positive way can be triggering, we also find it can be healing. Being the adult you needed growing up is a powerfully transformative experience.

How do I deal with a co-parent or other family member who isn't sex positive, and who doesn't agree with me sharing this information with a child?

It can be tough to face criticism, pushback, or completely opposing values from other adults in your child's world. It happens often with non-sex positive issues, but often can feel magnified when the topic relates to sex.

Some ways you can navigate the situation:

- If it feels safe for you to talk with the other adult, use communication that's focused on both people listening to understand versus respond. Talk through your different approaches, express any concerns or misunderstandings, with the hopes of finding common ground or new agreements.

- Be clear about what is in your sphere of influence versus control. It's not realistic to think that we can change another person's values or way of thinking about a topic, so it's not the best use of our energy to try. We can be of influence by living our truth or sharing knowledge. Knowing the difference can shift how much energy we put into discussions with or expectations of others.

- Be clear about your 'why'. Why is it important that you teach certain topics to your child or that you're preparing them with certain skills and knowledge? When we are clear about our 'why', we are better able to stand firm in the face of opposition.

- Know that it can be valuable for a child to experience different perspectives. It can help them as they are developing their own unique values.

- If the differing values include any concerns for the child's safety, be sure to maintain documentation of what you are observing, report if needed, or seek legal counsel and support.

- If the child is old enough, bring the issue out in the open. See what they think about the differing values and be open to hearing their own opinions without it being about choosing sides. Share with them your why, and what you hope for in the way you're choosing to parent them. Create space for them to share any impacts they may be experiencing related to the disagreements.

Q *How do I get my child to not talk about this stuff at school, without sounding like I'm shaming them?*

It's not uncommon for children to share with others the things that they're learning. Sexual health topics are definitely no exception. Because these discussions can be highly stigmatized and taboo, it can leave some parents feeling worried about getting a call from school or being confronted by another adult about what their child is sharing with other kids.

The reality is that we cannot control what our children may say or how they interact with others, especially when it's happening outside of our presence, but we can definitely equip them with guidance and context that helps them make an informed decision about when the best times and people are, or are not, to talk to about these topics.

To be proactive when talking with preschool and elementary aged kids, add language such as this within your sexual health talks:

> *"I'm really happy we get to talk about these things together. It's our special time, and it's important that we let other kids have time like this with their grownups. This means that we don't tell these facts to our friends or at school. Families can have different beliefs or different ways they want to share these talks together, so we want to respect that. Do you think you can keep that in mind? If a friend has a question about their body or about sex, let them know they should talk with their trusted adult."*

If you do receive a call or get notified that something was said by your child, try not to react from a place of shame. Punishing them is not the answer. The fact that they shared conversations with others is a sign that they are learning from your talks, they're engaged, and may just need a gentle reminder of where the boundaries should be while they're still young and learning.

TRUSTED SEXUAL HEALTH RESOURCES

Visit us online at sexpositivefamilies.com for more great resources to support the talks at every age and stage.

AMAZE
amaze.org
Engaging, inclusive animated videos and digital content on sexual health topics made for parents, children, and teens

BEDSIDER
bedsider.org
Birth control and contraception methods support and information

COLAGE
colage.org
National youth-driven network of people with LGBTQ+ parents offering workshops, conferences, resources, and support for rainbow families

COMMON SENSE MEDIA
commonsensemedia.org
Media literacy education, resources, and reviews for all types of media and programming relevant to kids of all ages and families

CYBERWISE
cyberwise.org
Resources and information about digital citizenship, internet safety, security, privacy, cyberbullying, sexting, and more to help kids embrace technology safely and wisely

GENDER SPECTRUM
genderspectrum.org
Comprehensive collection of research, resources, and stories to help any parent, caregiver, or professional learn more about gender diversity

HUMAN RIGHTS CAMPAIGN
hrc.org
LGBTQ+ rights and advocacy organization with resources for LGBTQ+ folx, queer youth, parents, and allies

INTERACT
interactadvocates.org
Advocacy and education organization in support of the human rights of children born with intersex traits

KIDSHEALTH
kidshealth.org
Child development information and resources, including sexual health in childhood

LOVE IS RESPECT
loveisrespect.org
Resources and education to empower youth to prevent and end dating abuse and intimate partner violence

PFLAG
pflag.org
Organization supporting parents, families, and allies with people who are LGBTQ+, with over 400 chapters nationwide

PLANNED PARENTHOOD
plannedparenthood.org
Sexual health resources, medical care, and education including Roo, a live chatbot available to answer sex ed questions from youth

PUT A CUP IN IT
putacupinit.com
Menstrual health education and interactive tools to find a menstrual health product that is right for you

RAINN (RAPE ABUSE INCEST NATIONAL NETWORK)
rainn.org
Education, advocacy, and resources for sexual abuse prevention including the 24-hour National Sexual Assault Hotline at 1-800-656-4673

RESPECTABILITY
respectability.org/resources/sexual-education-resources
Sexuality education resources for young adults with developmental and intellectual disabilities

SCARLETEEN
scarleteen.com
Inclusive, comprehensive, supportive sexuality and relationship information for teens and emerging adults

SEX ETC
sexetc.org
Comprehensive sexual health information for teens and emerging adults

SIECUS (SEXUALITY INFORMATION & EDUCATION COUNCIL OF THE UNITED STATES)
siecus.org
Sexuality education advocacy, research, and resources

STOP IT NOW!
stopitnow.org
Child sexual abuse prevention education, advocacy, and resources for families

THE TREVOR PROJECT
thetrevorproject.org
Crisis intervention services and supportive resources for LGBTQ+ youth and their families

GLOSSARY OF TERMS

Definitions can provide helpful examples and context as you learn about sexual health topics. When it comes to identity terms, remember that people get to define their own identity and experiences, what it means to them, and no one should ever be forced to define or label themselves to others. For a more expansive glossary, check out the resources available through sites like **scarleteen.com**, **hrc.org**, and **plannedparenthood.org.**

Agender (or genderless)—someone who does not identify with a gender. Some agender people use the term gender neutral or neutrois, some define their gender as unknown or not definable, and some agender people do not care about gender as a label.

Aromantic—someone who experiences little to no romantic attraction

Asexual—also known as "Ace" or "Aces" - Someone who experiences little or no sexual attraction, or who experiences attraction but doesn't feel the need to act out that attraction sexually. Asexual people can also identify in many other ways.

Barrier Method—a method of contraception that works by creating a barrier that does not allow sperm to reach an ovum. Barrier methods also can protect against the transmission of some sexually transmitted infections. Examples of barrier methods include internal condoms, external condoms, and dental dam

Bigender—someone who identifies with two genders

Binary—the belief that gender identity has only two distinct, opposite, and disconnected forms. Viewing gender as binary, is a belief that only men and women, male and female identities exist

Bisexual—sexual or romantic attraction toward others that is not limited to people of one gender

Cisgender—someone whose gender aligns within what is typically associated with their sex assigned at birth

Demisexual—someone who only experiences sexual attraction once they form an emotional connection with someone else

Dental Dam—a rectangular shaped sheet of latex or polyurethane that's used to protect against skin-to-skin contact or exchange of bodily fluids during oral sex on a vulva or anus. Dental dams are not commonly sold in stores, like external condoms, and can sometimes be found for free at sexual health clinics. Dental dams can be made easily though using an external condom and the following steps:

- Remove the external condom from its packaging. You can choose to use an unlubricated or lubricated condom, whichever you prefer.

- While the condom is still rolled, cut off the tip. You should be left with a ring-like shape.

- Cut a straight line through one side of the ring-like shape.

- Unroll the condom, and it should expand to a larger rectangle. This is your DIY dental dam!

Emotional Attraction—a feeling of deep connection to another person, with or without physical elements of attraction

Fallopian Tubes—the passages through which the ova (eggs) travel to the uterus

Gender Expression—the physical representation of a person's gender through things like their clothing choices, hair, or personal style. From a binary lens, it can relate to how feminine or masculine a person presents, but it can be a mix or neither of these. Examples of terms related to gender expression are feminine, masculine, androgynous, neutral, conforming, and nonconforming

Gender Identity—how someone thinks of or identifies themselves relative to gender. Examples are girl/woman, boy/man, femme, transgender, nonbinary, genderfluid, and genderqueer

Gender Nonconforming—someone whose gender identity and/or gender expression does not conform to the cultural or social expectations of gender. This can be an umbrella term for many identities including, but not limited to genderfluid, gender-expansive, and gender nonbinary

Gender Norms—constructed "rules" or ideas about the way members of certain genders "should" look and behave

Gender Pronouns—words that refer to who a person is talking to or talking about. For example: she/her/hers/herself; they/them/theirs/themself; ze/zir/zirs/zirself; and he/him/his/himself. A person determines which pronouns they identify with and it does not always correlate with a person's gender. Using someone's correct pronouns is a basic way to show respect for another person

Genderfluid—someone whose gender identity and/or expression varies and is not attached to one gender

Genderqueer—someone whose gender identity and/or expression is fluid and can fall between, outside of, or within both binary woman/man identities

Heteronormative—a worldview that elevates heterosexuality, the gender binary, and social norms related to heterosexuality, as normal or preferred

Intersex—a person that is born with genitals, chromosome patterns, internal organs, or hormone levels that fall outside of what's typically categorized as female or male. Because of these varying factors, that aren't always visible at birth, a person may not learn they are intersex until puberty or later in life or may never find this out about themselves.

LGBTQ+—an acronym that commonly stands for lesbian, gay, bisexual, transgender, and queer or questioning. The plus can be used to represent the expansive spectrum of identities and orientations

Menstruation—the shedding from the uterus of the thick endometrial lining that develops during ovulation

Misgendering—using language toward or to describe a transgender person, that doesn't align with their affirmed gender. For example, calling a transgender woman "he" or "him"

Ova—(singular ovum) the cells located in the ovaries of a person with a uterus, which contain half of what is needed genetically to create new life

Ovaries—two almond-shaped organs in the body of a person with a uterus where the ova are stored

Pangender—someone whose identity consists of all or many gender identities and expressions

Pansexual—someone who experiences emotional, romantic, or sexual attraction to people of any gender

Penis—an external organ made of erectile tissue that consists of two parts—the shaft and the glans (the tip, sometimes called the head)- and can transfer urine, sperm, and semen

Physical Attraction—a part of sexual identity often representing a draw or desire toward another person in a sexual or physical way

Queer—a term used to express fluid identities and orientations. In the past, queer was a negative or pejorative term for people who are gay, and thus it is sometimes disliked. The term is increasingly being used to describe all identities and politics that go against normative beliefs. The term is valued by many LGBTQ+ people for its defiance and sense of community

Sex Assigned at Birth— also referred to as biological sex- a label given when a person is born, that's often based on an assessment of their external genitals. Examples of these terms are female, male, and intersex

Sex Positive—an open, affirming, and judgment-free attitude toward human sexuality and sex that regards all consensual experiences as fundamentally healthy

Sexually Transmitted Infection (STI)—an infection caused by a bacterium, parasite, or virus that is passed from one person to another person through sexual contact. Examples include gonorrhea, herpes simplex 1 or 2 (oral or genital, respectively), human papillomavirus (HPV), chlamydia, syphilis, human immunodeficiency virus (HIV), and trichomoniasis.

Sperm—the cell produced in the testicles that contains half of what is needed genetically to create new life

Testicles—oval-shaped organs that produce sperm and testosterone

Transition—a term sometimes used to refer to the process— social, legal, and/or medical—one goes through to discover and/or affirm one's gender identity. This may, but does not always, include taking hormones; having surgeries; and changing names, pronouns, identification documents, and more. Many individuals choose not to or are unable to transition for a wide range of reasons both within and beyond their control. A trans person does not have to experience such transitions in order to identify as transgender

Transgender (trans)— someone who identifies with a gender that is different from the sex they were assigned at birth

Uterus—the internal organ, about the size of a pear, where endometrial lining can develop during menstrual cycles and where a fertilized ovum can develop into a fetus

Vagina—the internal muscular tube, of about 3 to 5 inches in length, that leads from the cervix to the outside of the body

Values—a person's principles or standards of behavior; one's judgment of what is important in their life

Vulva—the external genitalia that includes parts such as the mons pubis, inner and outer labia, glans clitoris, urethral opening, and vaginal opening

ABOUT THE AUTHOR

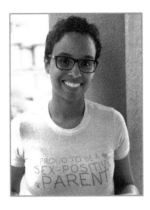

Melissa Pintor Carnagey (she or they) is a Black, Puerto Rican, and Mexican sexuality educator and licensed social worker based in Austin, Texas. Melissa launched Sex Positive Families in June 2017, inspired by the belief that all children deserve holistic, comprehensive, and shame-free sexuality education to live informed, empowered, and safer lives. She is confident that the work starts in homes with families and has seen the power of sex positive parenting thrive within her own life raising three young people, one who is now an adult.

Melissa's professional experience spans over a decade in the field of sexual health, having taught comprehensive sexuality education in schools, authored curricula, and worked within HIV/AIDS case management and prevention at both nonprofit and state government levels.

The work of Sex Positive Families has been featured in media such as *HuffPost, Parents Magazine, Mashable, ScaryMommy,* and *Mother Magazine.* Melissa has also collaborated with organizations such as *Advocates for Youth, AMAZE, Planned Parenthood Federation of America,* and *SIECUS* on projects that promote comprehensive, inclusive, consent-conscious, and pleasure-positive sexuality education for youth and families. With over 150,000 followers worldwide (@sexpositive_families), Sex Positive Families' presence and impact have made it a leading resource supporting parents on the path of raising sexually healthy children.

To learn more about Sex Positive Families and connect with resources to support your family, visit sexpositivefamilies.com.

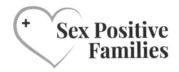

CPSIA information can be obtained
at www.ICGtesting.com
Printed in the USA
LVHW070733100123
736831LV00009B/205